BREAKING THE CRISIS ON LIPOEDEMA

Transform Your Life, A Comprehensive Guide To Understanding, Managing, For Overcoming Adiposalgia Challenges To Embrace Healing And Wellness

DR. RUNDELL MEEHAN

ABOUT THIS BOOK

"Breaking the Crisis on Lipoedema" is an indispensable resource that addresses a significant medical issue often overlooked in mainstream healthcare.

This book begins with a comprehensive introduction, providing readers with a foundational understanding of lipoedema, a condition characterized by an abnormal accumulation of fat cells in certain areas of the body, typically the legs and buttocks.

By delving into the historical perspectives and prevalence demographics, this book illuminates the urgency of ending the crisis surrounding lipoedema.

The table of contents outlines a structured approach to tackling the complexities of lipoedema. The chapters are meticulously organized, starting with consciousness and instruction, moving through diagnosis and medical assessment, lifestyle management, treatment options, living with lipoedema, research and innovations, healthcare systems, and concluding with global perspectives. Each chapter serves as a building block, systematically addressing various aspects of the condition, from its anatomical and physiological underpinnings to its psychosocial impacts, treatment modalities, and global implications.

One of this book's notable strengths lies in its emphasis on early diagnosis and holistic treatment approaches. By highlighting the importance of early detection, this book underscores the potential for better treatment outcomes and improved quality of life for patients. Furthermore, it provides a comprehensive overview of conservative and surgical interventions, empowering both patients and healthcare professionals with a range of options for managing lipoedema.

Moreover, "Breaking the Crisis on Lipoedema" goes beyond individual treatment strategies to address broader systemic issues within healthcare systems worldwide. Chapters dedicated to healthcare systems and global perspectives shed light on the challenges faced by patients in accessing appropriate care and advocate for improved awareness, education, and collaboration among stakeholders.

Overall, "Breaking the Crisis on Lipoedema" serves as a pivotal resource for patients, caregivers, and healthcare professionals alike, offering invaluable insights into a complex and often misunderstood condition. Through its meticulous research, comprehensive content, and impassioned advocacy, this book is poised to drive meaningful change in the understanding, diagnosis, and management of lipoedema on a global scale.

DISCLAIMER

This book is meant to give basic information and instructional material about health issues.

The information provided here is not meant to diagnose, treat, cure, or prevent any illness or medical condition.

It is not an alternative to professional medical advice, diagnosis, or treatment. If you have any concerns about a medical issue or your own or others' health and welfare, always see your physician or another trained health expert.

The author and publisher of this book have taken every effort to ensure that the material presented is correct and current at the time of publishing. They do not, however, make any explicit or implied representations or guarantees regarding the completeness, accuracy, reliability, appropriateness, or availability of the material provided herein.

Any reliance on such material is solely at your own risk.

The author and publisher do not promote or suggest any persons, goods, websites, organizations, or other names mentioned or referenced in this book. All such references are provided for informative reasons only.

Furthermore, the author and publisher are not responsible for any direct, indirect, consequential, or incidental damages or losses resulting from the use of the information included in this book. This includes, but is not limited to, mistakes, omissions, inaccuracies, and any results that occur from the use of the information given.

By reading this book, you indicate that you have read, understood, and accept the conditions of this disclaimer. If you do not agree to these conditions, do not use or depend on the information provided here. Before changing your diet, exercise routine, medication, or medical treatment plan, always speak with a trained healthcare expert.

Table of Contents

INTRODUCTION

Adipose tissue abnormally accumulates in the lower limbs of people with lipoedema, a chronic and progressive disorder that can also affect the upper limbs. It is often misinterpreted and misdiagnosed, which causes severe physical and mental hardships for those who are impacted. Raising awareness, advancing accurate diagnosis, and advocating for practical management techniques are all necessary to end the lipoedema crisis and improve the lives of those who suffer from it.

Understanding Lipoedema

The abnormal and disproportionate buildup of fat in particular body parts, usually the thighs, hips, buttocks, and occasionally the arms, is known as lipoedema. Lipoedema fat is unresponsive to diet and exercise, in contrast to general obesity. It causes a noticeable "bracelet" effect at the ankles and wrists and is characterized by a symmetrical distribution. It usually spares the hands and feet.

Defining Lipoedema

Because lipoedema and obesity are similar conditions, lipoedema is frequently misdiagnosed or disregarded. The main characteristics include easy bruising, discomfort, and exaggerated fat deposition. Common symptoms include pain and discomfort. Over time, lipoedema may cause joint and mobility problems. The majority of patients are female, and the onset of the condition is frequently associated with hormonal changes like puberty, pregnancy, or menopause.

Historical Perspectives

In the past, there has been a lack of understanding about lipoedema, leading to persistent misconceptions. The earliest known case occurred in the United States in the 1940s, but it wasn't until much later that scientists began to identify and investigate the illness in greater detail. Delays in diagnosis and ineffective management techniques have been caused by a lack of knowledge and a paucity of research.

Prevalence And Demographics

Females are more likely to suffer from lipoedema; estimates place the global incidence of the condition at up to 11%. Due to a lack of knowledge among medical professionals, the condition is frequently underdiagnosed, and its prevalence may be higher than previously thought. Hormonal factors and genetic predisposition are thought to be involved, though the precise cause is still unknown. The psychological effects of lipoedema, such as problems with body image and mental health, highlight the necessity of managing the condition holistically.

Ending The Lipoedema Crisis

1. Consciousness and Instruction:
Raising awareness among patients, healthcare providers, and the general public is essential to enhancing lipoedema early diagnosis and detection.

• Educational initiatives may assist debunk misconceptions about the illness and advance knowledge of its psychological and physical effects.

2. Investigation and Prognosis:

• Supporting studies to learn more about the causes and development of lipoedema.

• Creating diagnostic criteria and instruments that are more precise to support early diagnosis and intervention.

3. Holistic Methods of Treatment:

• Putting into practice interdisciplinary therapy strategies that deal with lipoedema's psychological as well as physical components.

• Giving patients access to specialist medical treatment, such as compression therapy, physical therapy, and counseling.

4. Assistance Networks:

• Creating support groups where people with lipoedema may communicate and exchange tips, coping mechanisms, and experiences.

• Promoting the creation of patient advocacy organizations to strengthen the voice of impacted parties and influence legislative reforms.

5. Training for Healthcare Professionals:

• Including lipoedema knowledge in medical school curricula and healthcare professionals' ongoing education initiatives.

• Ensuring that medical professionals have the tools necessary to identify and treat lipoedema effectively in their practices.

In summary, a comprehensive strategy including awareness, research, diagnosis, and holistic treatment approaches is needed to solve the lipoedema epidemic. Enhancing awareness of lipoedema and encouraging cooperation between researchers, advocacy organizations, and medical professionals may help improve the quality of life for those who suffer from this illness.

CHAPTER 1

Anatomy And Physiology Of Lipoedema

The abnormal and excessive buildup of fat, usually in the lower limbs, is the hallmark of lipoedema, a chronic illness that often causes discomfort, swelling, and reduced mobility. It is essential to comprehend the anatomy and physiology of lipoedema in order to effectively treat and resolve the crisis that this illness is connected with.

Adipose Tissue Overview

The tissue called adipose tissue, or fat, is essential to the functioning of the human body. It performs the roles of an organ cushion, heat insulator, and energy store.

However, the distribution of adipose tissue becomes abnormal in lipoedematous patients, affecting mostly the lower limbs. In contrast to normal weight growth, lipoedema fat often defies conventional diet and exercise regimens.

Asymmetrical and disproportionate distribution of the fat deposition gives lipoedema its distinctive look. A person with lipoedema may suffer pain and discomfort due to increased pressure on nearby tissues, blood vessels, and nerves as a result of this abnormal fat accumulation.

Lymphatic System And Its Role

As an essential part of the body's circulatory system, the lymphatic system helps the immune system, maintains fluid balance, and filters pollutants. The lymphatic system is weakened in lipoedema, which exacerbates the buildup of fluid in the afflicted regions.

Edema, or swelling, in the lower limbs, is a result of poor lymphatic drainage in lipoedema. This ongoing swelling has the potential to worsen over time and cause other issues including fibrosis and heightened infection susceptibility. Comprehending and tackling the lymphatic aspect of lipoedema is essential in mitigating the crisis and enhancing the general well-being of those impacted.

Genetic Factors In Lipoedema

The development of lipoedema is significantly influenced by genetic factors. Studies have shown a propensity to run in families, indicating a hereditary susceptibility to the illness. Evidence points to a hereditary component, albeit the exact genetic pathways are yet unknown.

Comprehending the genetic underpinnings of lipoedema may facilitate the development of tailored therapeutic approaches and timely treatments. Finding certain genetic markers linked to lipoedema might help develop tailored treatments and prevention measures for those who are more susceptible because of their family history.

In summary, resolving the crisis related to lipoedema requires a thorough grasp of the anatomy and physiology of the illness. Identifying the abnormal distribution of adipose tissue, treating lymphatic dysfunction, and determining the underlying genetic causes are essential stages in creating efficient treatment plans and enhancing the general quality of life for lipoedema patients. This information serves as the basis for further chapters that explore lipoedema diagnosis, treatment, and cutting-edge therapies.

CHAPTER 2

Signs And Symptoms

A chronic illness called lipoedema is characterized by excessive fat buildup, usually in the lower limbs, which results in an unnaturally uncomfortable and disproportionate body form. Comprehending the indications and manifestations of lipoedema is imperative for prompt identification and efficient management. Three main topics are covered in depth in this chapter: Differential Diagnosis, Progressive Symptoms, and Early Signs of Lipoedema.

Early Signs Of Lipoedema

1. One Leg on Both Sides:

• Bilateral limbs are often affected symmetrically by lipoedema. Its characteristic bilateral participation sets it apart from other diseases.

2. Disproportionate build-up of fat

• An abnormal build-up of fat that gives the body a disproportionate look about the upper body is one of the early indicators. The hips, thighs, buttocks, and even the lower legs are where this adipose tissue accumulation is most often seen.

3. Simplebruising and Sensitivity:

• Even with minimal injuries, people with lipoedema may bruise easily, and the afflicted regions may be painful to the touch. This is explained by the adipose tissue's enhanced blood vessel fragility.

4. Soreness or Unease:

• Pain may not necessarily accompany early-stage lipoedema, although discomfort is a possibility, particularly while standing or walking for extended periods. The degree of discomfort may increase as the illness worsens.

5. Preserving Foot Health:
• Usually, lipoedema spares the feet, in contrast to other disorders that cause

swelling in the legs. It may be distinguished from lymphedema by the characteristic "cuff" impression that is often created when the swelling ends at the ankle.

Progressive Symptoms

1. Deteriorating Disproportion

• As the excessive fat buildup worsens over time, the difference between the upper and lower bodies becomes more and more apparent.

2. heightened susceptibility to pressure

• The afflicted regions can become more sensitive to pressure; pain can arise from even the slightest touch or pressure from clothes. Patients often report this increased sensitivity as a throbbing or scorching feeling.

3. Mobility Difficulties:

• As lipoedema worsens, the weight and bulk of the lower limbs may rise, limiting movement. For those who are impacted, this may hurt everyday activities and lower their overall quality of life.

4. Psychosocial Repercussions:

• The cosmetic alterations brought on by lipoedema may have serious psychological ramifications. Patients may suffer from mental anguish, problems with their bodies, and a general decline in well-being.

Differential Diagnosis

1. Edema lymphatic:

• Because of the swelling in the legs, lymphedema and lipoedema are often mistaken. Nonetheless, lipoedema may be distinguished from lymphedema by the preservation of the feet and the absence of pitting edema.

2. Overweight:

• Although lipoedema is characterized by abnormal fat buildup, it is important to distinguish it from obesity in general. This differentiation may be made easier with the help of the distinctive disproportionate distribution of fat and sensitivity to touch.

3. The insufficiency of veins

Leg swelling may be brought on by chronic venous insufficiency; however, this condition usually affects the lower leg and is accompanied by additional symptoms such as varicose veins. Conversely, lipoedema mainly affects the areas of the upper legs.

4. Additional Lipodystrophies

• There may be some parallels between lipoedema and rare diseases like Dercum's disease or lipohypertrophy. A thorough assessment is required to differentiate between these circumstances.

Identifying lipoedema early on and differentiating it from other related disorders are essential for creating a successful treatment strategy. Healthcare practitioners may lessen the burden of lipoedema on patients' lives by diagnosing and intervening early with the help of the signs and symptoms covered in this chapter.

CHAPTER 3

Diagnosis And Medical Assessment

Chronic lipoedema is defined by abnormal fat buildup, usually in the lower limbs, which causes discomfort, swelling, and a major reduction in the quality of life for those who have it. To successfully manage and end the lipoedema crisis, a prompt and precise diagnosis is essential. The diagnostic procedure and medical evaluation are the main topics of Chapter 3, which emphasizes the significance of early diagnosis.

Clinical Evaluation

1. History of the patient:

• Start by taking a thorough patient history that includes information about the patient's family history, symptoms, and lifestyle choices.

• Examine the beginning and development of symptoms, keeping an eye out for any discomfort, soreness, or limb form changes.

2. Physical Assessment:

• Perform a comprehensive physical examination, noting skin texture, nodule presence, and the distribution of adipose tissue.

• Determine the degree of discomfort and edema, as well as any functional impairment.

• Distinguish lipoedema from illnesses like obesity or lymphedema that might exhibit symptoms that are similar to lipoedema.

3. Classification of Clinical Practices:

• Apply known clinical criteria, such as the Stemmer sign and water displacement tests, to categorize lipoedema phases.

• Take into account the most current revisions to the criteria and standards to improve diagnostic accuracy.

Imaging Techniques

1. Imaging using ultrasound:

• Use high-resolution ultrasonography to examine the properties of fat deposits and see the subcutaneous tissue.

• Recognize certain characteristics that may help diagnose lipoedema, such as fluid buildup and hyperechoic septa.

2. MRIs, or magnetic resonance imaging:

• To get a thorough evaluation of the distribution of fat and the involvement of nearby tissues, think about MRI.

• A more thorough knowledge of tissue composition is provided by MRI, which helps with therapy planning and differential diagnosis.

• By measuring the distribution of fat and lean tissue, DEXA scans may help with objective measures and treatment response monitoring.

Importance Of Early Diagnosis

1. Better Results from the Treatment:

• Prompt diagnosis enhances the efficacy of treatment plans by enabling the necessary therapeutic measures to be started right away.

• Treating lipoedema early on will help avoid or lessen consequences including psychological anguish and subsequent lymphedema.

2. Improved Standard of Living:

• A prompt diagnosis and course of treatment may reduce pain and improve mobility while also increasing the patient's quality of life and symptom relief.

• Prompt treatment may help stop lipoedema from developing into more severe stages.

3. Patient Empowerment and Education:

• Early diagnosis helps medical professionals inform patients about the illness, which promotes a better comprehension of lifestyle changes and self-management techniques.

• Patients who feel empowered are more likely to take an active role in their treatment, which improves results over time.

4. Expense-effectiveness:

• Early diagnosis may reduce the need for significant treatments and interventions that are necessary at later stages, which might lead to more affordable healthcare delivery.

In summary, Chapter 3 emphasizes the need for a comprehensive clinical examination and the use of cutting-edge imaging methods, which is crucial in breaking the crisis related to lipoedema. People with lipoedema who get an early diagnosis not only benefit from better treatment results but also have greater overall quality of life. Using these diagnostic techniques in clinical practice adds to a thorough and successful lipoedema therapy plan.

CHAPTER 4

Psychosocial Impact

A chronic illness called lipoedema is characterized by an abnormal build-up of fat, usually in the lower limbs, which causes discomfort, swelling, and other associated symptoms. Although lipoedema's physical effects are well-established, its psychological effects should also be taken into consideration.

People who have lipoedema often have emotional difficulties, battle concerns related to their bodies and self-worth, and use a variety of coping techniques to manage the intricacies of this illness.

Emotional Challenges

1. Anxiety and Depression: Having a long-term illness like lipoedema may be emotionally draining. Depression and anxiety may be exacerbated by the ongoing pain, discomfort, and possible restrictions on everyday activities. Having doubts about how the illness will proceed and how it will affect one's quality of life may make these emotional difficulties much worse.

2. Chronic stress and frustration may result from managing the physical symptoms of lipoedema, such as pain and swelling. Frustration might also result from the difficulties in controlling the effects on day-to-day living and finding efficient treatment choices.

The emotional toll may damage relationships with others and impair general well-being.

Body Image And Self-Esteem

1. **Unfavorable Body Image:** Lipoedema often causes an uneven distribution of fat, especially in the lower limbs. Because of this physical attribute, people may have a poor body image because they feel self-conscious about how they look. Negative thoughts regarding one's physique might also arise as a result of society's expectations of beauty.

2. **Effect on Self-esteem:** Self-esteem may be greatly impacted by the outward manifestations of lipoedema as well as

social assumptions and judgments. People may internalize the ideals of beauty set by society, which may result in a lower feeling of self-worth. For people with lipoedema to cultivate a good self-image, it is important to address certain difficulties related to self-esteem.

Coping Mechanisms

1. **Social Support:** To manage the psychological effects of lipoedema, it is critical to establish a robust support network. Encouragement, understanding, and emotional support may be obtained from friends, family, and support groups. Within the lipoedema group, shared experiences may lessen feelings of loneliness and provide a sense of acceptance.

2. Therapeutic Interventions: Individuals may learn coping mechanisms to manage the emotional effects of lipoedema by seeking professional psychological assistance, such as therapy or counseling. Counselors may provide a secure environment for discussing and resolving the emotional difficulties brought on by having a chronic illness.

3. Education and Advocacy: Providing people with information on lipoedema will help them cope better. A feeling of agency and control may be obtained by being aware of the illness, and the available treatments, and establishing contact with advocacy organizations. Education may also support increased awareness and assist dispel social stigmas.

4. Healthy Lifestyle Options: Adopting a holistic approach to health, which takes into account the restrictions of lipoedema and includes regular exercise and a balanced diet, may have a good effect on one's physical and emotional well-being. Making healthy lifestyle choices enhances resilience and self-control in general.

The psychosocial effects of lipoedema include identifying and comprehending the emotional difficulties, problems with body image, and self-esteem concerns that people may have. The adoption of efficacious coping strategies, including education, counseling, social support, and healthy lifestyle choices, is crucial in resolving the lipoedema crisis and improving the general quality of life.

CHAPTER 5

Lifestyle Management

A chronic illness called lipoedema is characterized by an abnormal build-up of fat, usually in the lower limbs, which causes discomfort, edema, and limited movement. In order to overcome the lipoedema crisis, lifestyle management is essential for assisting patients in managing their illness and enhancing their general quality of life. Three major facets of lifestyle management are covered in this chapter: the importance of weight control, exercise and physical activity, and nutrition guidelines.

Nutrition Guidelines

Nutrition is essential for the management of lipoedema since food choices affect fluid balance, inflammation, and general health. Think about the following dietary recommendations:

1. **Anti-Inflammatory Diet:** Place a focus on foods that have anti-inflammatory qualities, such as whole grains, fruits, vegetables, and fatty seafood that are high in omega-3 fatty acids. Reduce your consumption of sugary snacks, processed meals, and saturated fats.

2. **Hydration:** Maintaining fluid balance requires enough hydration. People who have lipoedema should be encouraged to drink

enough water throughout the day since dehydration may make swelling worse.

3. Consumption of Salt: Consuming too much salt might cause fluid retention. Advocate for a diet low in sodium and stress the use of spices and herbs rather than salt for seasoning.

4. Encourage the consumption of balanced meals that include a variety of carbs, healthy fats, and protein. This aids in controlling blood sugar levels and deters overindulgence in food.

5. Meal Timing: To control metabolism and energy levels, encourage regular, balanced meal timings. Encourage them not to miss meals since erratic eating habits might throw off their hormone balance.

Exercise And Physical Activity

Exercise regularly is essential for reducing the symptoms of lipoedema, boosting circulation, and increasing general mobility. Customize workout suggestions according to each person's ability and preferences:

1. **Low-Impact Exercises:** Choose low-impact activities like swimming, cycling, or walking since they are less taxing on the joints and aid in reducing swelling without putting too much pressure on them.

2. **Strength exercise:** To increase muscular tone, do mild resistances exercise. Enhancing the muscles around the impacted regions might provide further assistance to the lymphatic system.

3. Stretching activities are a good way to increase flexibility and joint range of motion. In this sense, yoga and pilates might be helpful.

4. Encourage people to progressively increase the time and intensity of their exercises by starting gently. Steer clear of overexertion to prevent symptoms from becoming worse.

5. Wearing compression clothing while exercising is advised to assist control of edema and provide extra support.

Importance Of Weight Management

Obesity does not cause lipoedema, however, being overweight may aggravate symptoms and reduce the impact of lifestyle changes.

Maintaining a healthy weight is essential for managing lipoedema and general health.

1. **Tailored Approach:** Acknowledge that people with lipoedema may not benefit from conventional weight-loss techniques. Rather than resorting to drastic diets, concentrate on making lifestyle modifications to reach and maintain a healthy weight.

2. **Healthy Eating Practices:** Encourage a long-term, well-rounded approach to nutrition. Promote portion management, mindful eating, and an emphasis on nutrient-dense meals.

3. **Collaborative Care:** Create a thorough weight-management strategy that is suited to the particular requirements of each person with lipoedema by collaborating with

medical specialists, such as physiotherapists and nutritionists.

4. Psychological Support: Recognize the emotional difficulties in managing weight when lipoedema is present. As part of the overall treatment plan, provide psychological assistance and think about including counseling or support groups.

To sum up, Chapter 5's discussion of lifestyle management is essential to resolving the lipoedema issue. Through proper diet, moderate physical exercise, and emphasis on weight control, people may improve their overall quality of life and effectively manage the symptoms of lipoedema. When paired with medical therapies, this all-encompassing approach may help provide a thorough and successful care plan for people with lipoedema.

CHAPTER 6

Treatment Options

A chronic illness called lipoedema is characterized by an abnormal build-up of fat, usually in the lower limbs, which causes discomfort, edema, and limited movement. Although lipoedema cannot be cured, several therapeutic options may help patients manage their symptoms and enhance their quality of life. This chapter explores the many techniques for treating lipoedema, including conservative measures, physical therapy, compression therapy, and surgical therapies such as liposuction and other operations.

Conservative Approaches

Whenever lipoedema symptoms are being managed, conservative measures are often the first line of defense. These tactics emphasize non-invasive methods and lifestyle adjustments to relieve pain and minimize edema.

Nutrition and Diet

A balanced, healthful diet is essential for those with lipoedema. Although the aberrant fat deposits that characterize lipoedema may not be directly targeted by weight reduction, keeping a healthy weight may assist manage general health and lessen the strain on the lymphatic system.

Frequent, low-impact physical activity is crucial for enhancing lymphatic flow and advancing general health. For those with lipoedema, exercises like swimming, walking, and light yoga might help control weight and reduce swelling.

Compression Therapy

Compression treatment is the application of external pressure and lymphatic system assistance via the use of specialized clothing, such as bandages or compression stockings. This lessens the pain and swelling brought on by lipoedema.

Stockings with Compression

The goal of graduated compression stockings is to provide maximum pressure at the ankles and progressively less pressure as they go up the thighs. Regularly using these stockings may help reduce symptoms and stop fluid accumulation.

Adhesion

Healthcare providers may use bandaging procedures to offer targeted compression and decrease edema in more severe situations. For this procedure to be used correctly, certain training is needed.

Physical Therapy

Physical therapy, which focuses on exercises and strategies to increase mobility, decrease discomfort, and improve general function, is essential in treating the symptoms of lipoedema.

Lymphatic Drainage by Hand (MLD)

The goal of MLD, a specific massage technique, is to increase lymphatic flow. To assist minimize swelling and pain, certified therapists circulate the lymphatic fluid with gentle, rhythmic motions.

Lymphatic Decongestive Therapy (DLT)
Combining many treatment modalities such as MLD, compression therapy, exercise, and skincare, DLT offers a holistic strategy.

It is often advised to use this combined strategy for those with advanced lipoedema.

Surgical Interventions

Surgical procedures become a feasible option to manage the abnormal fat deposits associated with lipoedema when conservative therapies are deemed ineffective.

Liposuction

One surgical technique for removing extra fat deposits is liposuction. Specialized methods like tumescent liposuction or water-assisted liposuction may be used in the context of lipoedema to target the afflicted regions and provide long-term relief.

Other Surgical Procedures

More involved surgical techniques, including lymphatic venous anastomosis (LVA) or debulking operations, could be explored in some circumstances. While LVA includes establishing connections between lymphatic arteries and veins to facilitate fluid outflow, debulking seeks to decrease the bulk of adipose tissue.

Lipoedema therapy is complex and often involves both conservative and surgical methods. The intensity of the symptoms, the unique features of each patient, and the advice of medical experts all influence the treatment decision. For lipoedema patients to benefit from improved overall health and management, a comprehensive and individualized strategy is essential.

CHAPTER 7

Living With Lipoedema

A persistent illness called lipoedema is characterized by an abnormal build-up of fat, mostly in the legs but sometimes occasionally in the arms. Physically and psychologically taxing, living with lipoedema may be difficult for those who must manage the condition's effects on day-to-day activities. This chapter examines several facets of having lipoedema, emphasizing patient viewpoints, the value of social networks, and the contribution of activism and education to ending the condition's crisis.

Patient Perspectives

To provide complete treatment and support, it is important to comprehend the experiences and viewpoints of those who are living with lipoedema. Physical difficulties that patients often experience, such as pain, swelling, and restricted movement, may have a serious negative influence on their quality of life. An additional layer of difficulty is the emotional toll that comes with managing a chronic ailment that may not be fully understood by the general population or even by certain healthcare experts.

1. Pain Control:
• Patients often experience pain related to lipoedema, which may range from mild

discomfort to excruciating agony. Investigating efficient pain relief techniques is crucial to enhancing the general health of lipoedema sufferers.

• To manage pain and increase mobility, physical therapy, compression treatment, and other non-pharmacological methods may be quite important.

2. Effect on the Mind:

• It's important to recognize the psychological effects of having a visible, often misdiagnosed illness like lipoedema. People may struggle with feelings of loneliness, despair, anxiety, and body image.

• It is essential to include mental health care in the entire treatment plan to assist patients in managing the emotional components of their illness.

Support Networks

Establishing and sustaining robust support systems is crucial for people with lipoedema. Support from medical experts, relatives, friends, and the larger community falls under this category.

1. Medical Practitioners:

• Patient and healthcare provider collaboration is essential. This comprises allied health workers as well as medical experts, including dietitians, physical therapists, and mental health counselors.

• Promoting a multidisciplinary approach to treatment guarantees that people with lipoedema get comprehensive care that meets their different requirements.

• The well-being of people with lipoedema may be greatly impacted by the support of friends and family. Teaching others in close circles about the illness promotes empathy and understanding.

• Help with everyday tasks or emotional support at trying times are examples of practical help that may make a big impact.

Advocacy And Awareness

Initiatives to raise awareness and advocate for change are essential to ending the lipoedema issue. This includes both patient advocacy on an individual basis and more general initiatives to raise public and professional awareness of the illness.

1. Advocacy for Patients:

• It's crucial to provide people with lipoedema the tools they need to advocate for themselves. This involves offering instruments and resources for self-advocacy, such as data about rights, therapies, and support systems.

• Encouraging patients to tell their tales may also help to dispel social stigmas and create a more accepting atmosphere.

• Raising public knowledge of lipoedema is essential to dispelling myths and fostering comprehension. To do this, public campaigns, educational programs, and media outreach may all be very important.

• Working together with legislators, patient advocacy groups, and healthcare organizations may help to further increase awareness about lipoedema.

• Education on lipoedema should be provided to medical professionals, including specialists and primary care doctors, to enhance timely diagnosis and effective treatment.

Within the medical community, publications, conferences, and continuing medical education programs may help spread current knowledge regarding lipoedema.

Managing physical and psychological difficulties, creating strong support systems, and promoting greater knowledge and comprehension are all necessary components of living with lipoedema. Lipoedema sufferers may help end the condition's crisis and enhance their overall quality of life by emphasizing patient viewpoints.

CHAPTER 8

Research And Innovations

A chronic illness called lipoedema is characterized by an abnormal build-up of fat, usually in the lower limbs, which causes discomfort, edema, and limited movement. Keeping up with the most recent findings and advancements in lipoedema research is an essential part of adopting a multifaceted strategy to address the situation. We explore the present status of research, new treatment options, and potential future paths in the area of lipoedema in this chapter.

Current Research

1. Studies in Genetics and Molecular Biology:

• Investigations into the genetic and molecular elements influencing the onset and course of lipoedema are still ongoing. Targeted therapy may become possible if the underlying genetic pathways are better understood.

• To learn more about the potential roles that certain gene expressions, hormone effects, and inflammatory pathways may have in the pathophysiology of lipoedema.

2. Technologies for Imaging:
The examination of lipoedema may now be done with more accuracy and detail because

of developments in imaging technologies like lymphoscintigraphy and magnetic resonance imaging (MRI). This aids in the comprehension of lymphatic malfunction and the distribution of adipose tissue.

• Personalized models of the afflicted limbs are being created using 3D imaging technology to help with treatment planning and monitoring.

3. Research on the Lymphatic System:

Research on the lymphatic system's involvement in lipoedema is ongoing. To lessen fluid buildup and enhance lymphatic function, researchers are looking at techniques to possibly alleviate symptoms.

The goal of the research is to create medications that target lymphatic veins and encourage lymphatic drainage.

4. Patient-Reported Results and Life Quality:

The effect of lipoedema on patients' quality of life is a topic of rising interest in research. This includes evaluating the condition's psychological effects, degree of discomfort, and functional restrictions.

• When developing therapy strategies that improve general well-being in addition to treating physical symptoms, patient-reported outcomes are crucial.

Emerging Therapies

• DLT is still the mainstay of lipoedema treatment, including manual lymphatic drainage, compression therapy, exercise, and skincare. These methods are being improved and optimized by ongoing study.

• The goal of innovations in compression apparel is to increase compliance and comfort via the use of cutting-edge materials and unique designs.

• The reduction of extra fat in lipoedema patients has been shown by liposuction, especially water-assisted liposuction.

To ascertain the safety and long-term effectiveness of these techniques, research is still being conducted.

• To treat lymphatic dysfunction, new surgical techniques such as vascularized lymph node transfer (VLNT) and lymphatic venous anastomosis (LVA) are being investigated.

3. Drug-Related Interventions:

The goal of current research is to find medications that may alter the underlying mechanisms causing lipoedema. This covers hormones, anti-inflammatory drugs, and possible medicines that target the metabolism of adipose tissue.

• Clinical studies are being undertaken to assess the effectiveness of drugs in lowering pain and inflammation as well as delaying the onset of lipoedema.

Future Directions

1. Precision Health Care:

• The discipline is moving toward individualized therapy plans that take into account patient traits such as genetic predispositions and unique symptom profiles.

• Interventions that are specifically designed to meet the requirements of each patient have the potential to be more successful and focused.

2. Digital Health Solutions:

• Digital health technologies, including wearables and mobile apps, may be integrated to improve patient self-management and provide medical professionals access to real-time data.

• Telemedicine platforms are becoming more and more significant, enabling lipoedema patients to get remote monitoring and consultations.

3. Research Collaboration Initiatives:

• Promoting cooperation between physicians, scientists, and patient advocacy organizations is essential to the advancement of lipoedema research. This kind of teamwork may hasten the application of scientific discoveries to therapeutic settings.

• By facilitating data exchange, international research networks may enable more diversified and sizable study populations.

In summary, resolving the lipoedema issue will need an ongoing dedication to research and innovation. Healthcare providers may improve the lives of lipoedema patients by remaining abreast of scientific developments and offering more individualized and effective therapies.

CHAPTER 9

Healthcare Systems And Lipoedema

Chronic and sometimes misdiagnosed, lipoedema is defined by abnormal fat buildup, usually in the lower limbs, which causes discomfort, swelling, and a reduced quality of life in those who have it. A thorough grasp of healthcare systems and their change is necessary to successfully diagnose, treat, and assist patients in the face of the lipoedema problem. This chapter explores the difficulties in providing lipoedema healthcare, the value of patient advocacy, and methods to increase treatment accessibility.

Challenges In Healthcare Delivery

1. Ignorance and incorrect diagnosis:

Lipoedema is often misdiagnosed or underdiagnosed, which results in insufficient or delayed therapy. Healthcare systems should place a high priority on educating medical personnel so they may identify and diagnose lipoedema early on.

2. Restricted Specialty Clinics and Physicians:

One factor adding to the difficulties patients confront is the lack of specialist clinics and medical professionals knowledgeable in lipoedema treatment. Improving patient outcomes will need educating medical experts to specialize in lipoedema treatment and expanding the number of clinics offering this kind of therapy.

3. Insufficient Guidelines for Treatment:

One major obstacle is the lack of detailed and consistent treatment recommendations for lipoedema. In order to provide evidence-based recommendations covering all facets of lipoedema treatment, from conservative approaches to surgical therapies, healthcare institutions must engage in research.

4. Budgetary Obstacles:

Patients may have to bear a heavy financial burden from the operations and treatments needed to address lipoedema. To lessen the financial burden on impacted people, healthcare systems should look at opportunities for government help, insurance, or financial aid.

5. Broken Care:

A multidisciplinary strategy is often necessary to treat lipoedema, comprising different medical specialists like surgeons, nutritionists, and lymphedema therapists. A comprehensive and successful treatment strategy depends on the integration and coordination of care across disciplines.

Patient Advocacy

1. Giving Patients Knowledge to Empower Them:

Patient advocacy is essential to ending the lipoedema epidemic. Patients may actively engage in their care and serve as their advocates when they are well informed about their disease, available treatments, and support resources.

2. Support Systems and Alliances:

Establishing and promoting networks and support groups dedicated to lipoedema enables sufferers to interact with others going through comparable struggles. These platforms let people feel connected, provide emotional support, and exchange insightful knowledge and life experiences.

3. Promoting Research Funding Advocacy:

Patients may lobby for more research funding to better understand the causes of lipoedema, provide better treatment choices, and eventually discover a solution with organizations and healthcare experts. Improved healthcare practices and results may result from more research.

Improving Access To Treatment

1. Training for Medical Professionals:

Healthcare organizations need to provide ongoing education initiatives for medical staff members to guarantee they remain current on advances in the study and management of lipoedema. Online courses, conferences, and workshops may all be used to give this instruction.

2. Services for Telehealth:
Access to lipoedema treatment may be enhanced by using telemedicine services, especially for patients who live in rural

regions or have mobility issues. Telehealth consultations may help with regular check-ins, direction, and continuous assistance.

3. Programs for Community Outreach:

Initiating community outreach initiatives may assist in locating instances of lipoedema that are not yet identified and informing the public about the illness. These initiatives may also act as a conduit for connecting patients with support services and other healthcare resources.

4. Working Together with Patient Advocacy Organizations:

To better understand the difficulties experienced by people with lipoedema, patient advocacy organizations and healthcare institutions should actively work together. Initiatives and policies focused on the needs of the patient may result from this partnership.

In summary, a multifaceted strategy including increased patient empowerment, treatment accessibility, and knowledge is needed to solve the lipoedema epidemic in healthcare systems. Healthcare systems may help people with lipoedema achieve better results and, in the end, live better lives by identifying and addressing these obstacles.

CHAPTER 10

Global Perspectives On Lipoedema

Globally, lipoedema—a chronic, misdiagnosed illness marked by abnormal fat buildup, mainly in the lower extremities—presents a major problem to patients and medical personnel. To address the problem surrounding lipoedema, we explore the worldwide views on the illness in this chapter, highlighting the significance of global awareness, variations in diagnosis and treatment, and cooperative efforts for research and education.

International Awareness

1. Absence of Acknowledgment:

Globally, lipoedema is still underdiagnosed and underrecognized. Increasing global awareness is essential for increasing the rate of early diagnosis, decreasing the number of misdiagnoses, and helping medical professionals get a better knowledge of the illness.

2. Advocacy for Patients:

The empowerment of lipoedema sufferers to speak out for themselves should be a global priority. Patient-led projects, public awareness efforts, and social media campaigns may help dispel the stigma attached to lipoedema and create a welcoming environment that promotes candid communication and information sharing.

3. Campaigns for Education:

Launching educational campaigns requires cooperation from international health agencies, patient advocacy groups, and healthcare organizations. These educational programs regarding lipoedema symptoms, risk factors, and therapies should be directed at both medical professionals and the general public.

Variances In Diagnosis And Treatment

1. Diagnostic Difficulties:

Because of differences in medical education, body image judgments, and awareness, diagnosing lipoedema may present particular difficulties in different geographical areas. Global efforts to standardize diagnostic criteria and enhance healthcare professional training are necessary to address these inequalities.

2. Disparities in Treatment:

Inequalities in access to and treatment choices may make the lipoedema issue worse. Developing and sharing evidence-based treatment recommendations should be the main goal of collaborative efforts to guarantee that patients everywhere have access to the right therapy, which includes psychiatric support, surgical treatments, and conservative therapies.

3. Cooperation in Research:

Research partnerships across international borders may be essential in identifying the genetic, environmental, and hormonal components that contribute to lipoedema. Collaborative clinical trials, multicenter investigations, and shared data may expedite the discovery of targeted medicines and enhance overall patient outcomes.

Collaborative Efforts For Research And Education

1. International Research Networks:

The creation of international research networks with specialists from different nations may help to share research results and expertise.

These networks may stimulate cooperative research, systematic reviews, and meta-analyses to improve our knowledge of lipoedema and direct the use of evidence-based medicine.

2. Instructional Plans:

International partnerships need to include academic establishments, cultivating the creation of training curricula tailored to the needs of healthcare practitioners dealing with lipoedema. This guarantees that medical professionals everywhere have the information and abilities required to properly identify and treat lipoedema.

3. Sharing of Resources:

Sharing instructional resources, such as guidelines, best practices, and informative materials, should be a part of collaborative initiatives. This interchange may contribute to the worldwide standardization of care by encouraging consistency in the diagnosis and management of lipoedema.

In conclusion, a coordinated international effort is needed to resolve the lipoedema epidemic. Increasing global awareness, resolving variations in diagnosis and treatment, and collaborating on research and education projects are crucial elements of a comprehensive plan to enhance the lives of people with this sometimes disregarded illness. We cannot improve global lipoedema patient outcomes, minimize treatment inequalities, or expand our knowledge without working together.

CONCLUSION

To sum up, combating the lipoedema epidemic calls for a multimodal strategy that includes education, prompt diagnosis, all-encompassing treatment plans, and continuing research. Patients with lipoedema, a chronic illness that is often misdiagnosed, have many difficulties, as does the healthcare system. We can enhance outcomes and the quality of life for people with lipoedema by treating several components of the disorder.

The most important thing to do is to increase awareness about lipoedema. Many people with lipoedema go untreated or are misdiagnosed, which causes symptoms to worsen and care to be delayed.

Patients, healthcare providers, and the general public should all be informed about the warning signs, symptoms, and implications of lipoedema. A greater understanding may result in an early diagnosis and prompt beginning of the right course of therapy.

One of the most important factors in ending the lipoedema crisis is early detection. Both the diagnostic criteria and the training of healthcare personnel to identify the illness should be widely distributed. This entails differentiating lipoedema using a mix of imaging techniques, patient history, and clinical examination from other disorders, such as obesity or lymphedema.

It is necessary to use comprehensive treatment options to address both the psychological and physical components of lipoedema. It is essential to use a multidisciplinary strategy that encompasses a range of healthcare experts, such as physiotherapists, dietitians, mental health specialists, and vascular specialists. To get the best results, surgical procedures like liposuction should be paired with conservative methods including compression therapy, manual lymphatic drainage, and exercise.

Research is essential to ending the lipoedema epidemic. Prevention and treatment advances may result from ongoing research into genetic variables, underlying causes, and prospective risk factors. To investigate novel therapy modalities and enhance already available therapies, clinical trials, and cooperative research projects are required.

Furthermore, for comprehensive therapy, treating the psychological components of lipoedema is essential. Patients often struggle with issues of self-worth, body image, and mental health. The general quality of life for people with lipoedema may be greatly improved by support groups, therapy, and educational initiatives.

In summary, healthcare providers, researchers, legislators, and the general public must work together to end the lipoedema issue. We can significantly improve the lives of individuals impacted by lipoedema by raising awareness, encouraging early diagnosis, putting thorough treatment plans into place, and furthering research. We can end the crisis cycle brought on by this often disregarded illness by working together and making a commitment to continued education and study.

THE END